This journal belongs to

____

____

____

Today's Goal

M T W T F **S** **S**

Muscle Group Focus ___________________ Weight ______ Date/Time ______

Stretch ◯   Warm-Up ___________________

Strength Training

Exercise		Set 1	Set 2	Set 3	Set 4	Set 5	Set 6
	Reps						
	Weight						
	Reps						
	Weight						
	Reps						
	Weight						
	Reps						
	Weight						
	Reps						
	Weight						
	Reps						
	Weight						
	Reps						
	Weight						
	Reps						
	Weight						
	Reps						
	Weight						
	Reps						
	Weight						

Cardio

Exercise	Calories	Distance	Time

Water Intake ___________________

Cooldown ___________________

Feeling ☆ ☆ ☆ ☆ ☆

Notes

Today's Goal

M · T · W · T · F · **S** · **S**

Muscle Group Focus ___________________________ Weight _______ Date/Time _______

Stretch ◯   Warm-Up ___________________________

Strength Training

Exercise		Set 1	Set 2	Set 3	Set 4	Set 5	Set 6
	Reps						
	Weight						
	Reps						
	Weight						
	Reps						
	Weight						
	Reps						
	Weight						
	Reps						
	Weight						
	Reps						
	Weight						
	Reps						
	Weight						
	Reps						
	Weight						
	Reps						
	Weight						
	Reps						
	Weight						

Cardio

Exercise	Calories	Distance	Time

Water Intake ___________________

Cooldown ___________________

Feeling ☆ ☆ ☆ ☆ ☆

Notes

Today's Goal

(M) (T) (W) (T) (F) **(S)** **(S)**

Muscle Group Focus ___________________ Weight ______ Date/Time ______

Stretch ◯   Warm-Up ___________________

Strength Training

Exercise		Set 1	Set 2	Set 3	Set 4	Set 5	Set 6
	Reps						
	Weight						
	Reps						
	Weight						
	Reps						
	Weight						
	Reps						
	Weight						
	Reps						
	Weight						
	Reps						
	Weight						
	Reps						
	Weight						
	Reps						
	Weight						
	Reps						
	Weight						
	Reps						
	Weight						

Cardio

Exercise	Calories	Distance	Time

Water Intake ___________________

Cooldown ___________________

Feeling ☆ ☆ ☆ ☆ ☆

Notes

Today's Goal

(M) (T) (W) (T) (F) (S) (S)

Muscle Group Focus ___________________________ Weight _________ Date/Time _________

Stretch ◯   Warm-Up ____

Strength Training

Exercise		Set 1	Set 2	Set 3	Set 4	Set 5	Set 6
	Reps						
	Weight						
	Reps						
	Weight						
	Reps						
	Weight						
	Reps						
	Weight						
	Reps						
	Weight						
	Reps						
	Weight						
	Reps						
	Weight						
	Reps						
	Weight						
	Reps						
	Weight						
	Reps						
	Weight						

Cardio

Exercise	Calories	Distance	Time

Water Intake _______________

Cooldown _______________

Feeling ☆ ☆ ☆ ☆ ☆

Notes

Today's Goal

M T W T F S S

Muscle Group Focus   Weight   Date/Time

Stretch ○   Warm-Up

Strength Training

Exercise		Set 1	Set 2	Set 3	Set 4	Set 5	Set 6
	Reps						
	Weight						
	Reps						
	Weight						
	Reps						
	Weight						
	Reps						
	Weight						
	Reps						
	Weight						
	Reps						
	Weight						
	Reps						
	Weight						
	Reps						
	Weight						
	Reps						
	Weight						
	Reps						
	Weight						

Cardio

Exercise	Calories	Distance	Time

Water Intake

Cooldown

Feeling ☆ ☆ ☆ ☆ ☆

Notes

Today's Goal

M T W T F S S

Muscle Group Focus ___________________ Weight _______ Date/Time _______

Stretch ◯ Warm-Up _______________________________

Strength Training

Exercise		Set 1	Set 2	Set 3	Set 4	Set 5	Set 6
	Reps						
	Weight						
	Reps						
	Weight						
	Reps						
	Weight						
	Reps						
	Weight						
	Reps						
	Weight						
	Reps						
	Weight						
	Reps						
	Weight						
	Reps						
	Weight						
	Reps						
	Weight						

Cardio

Exercise	Calories	Distance	Time

Water Intake _______

Cooldown _______

Feeling ☆ ☆ ☆ ☆ ☆

Notes

Today's Goal

Muscle Group Focus ___________ Weight _______ Date/Time _______

Stretch ◯   Warm-Up ___________

M T W T F **S** **S**

Strength Training

Exercise		Set 1	Set 2	Set 3	Set 4	Set 5	Set 6
	Reps						
	Weight						
	Reps						
	Weight						
	Reps						
	Weight						
	Reps						
	Weight						
	Reps						
	Weight						
	Reps						
	Weight						
	Reps						
	Weight						
	Reps						
	Weight						
	Reps						
	Weight						

Cardio

Exercise	Calories	Distance	Time

Water Intake ___________

Cooldown ___________

Feeling ☆ ☆ ☆ ☆ ☆

Notes

Today's Goal

Muscle Group Focus ______________________ Weight ______ Date/Time ______

Stretch ◯   Warm-Up ______________________

Strength Training

Exercise		Set 1	Set 2	Set 3	Set 4	Set 5	Set 6
	Reps						
	Weight						
	Reps						
	Weight						
	Reps						
	Weight						
	Reps						
	Weight						
	Reps						
	Weight						
	Reps						
	Weight						
	Reps						
	Weight						
	Reps						
	Weight						
	Reps						
	Weight						
	Reps						
	Weight						

Cardio

Exercise	Calories	Distance	Time

Water Intake ______________

Cooldown ______________

Feeling ☆ ☆ ☆ ☆ ☆

Notes

Today's Goal

(M) (T) (W) (T) (F) (S) (S)

Muscle Group Focus ___________________ Weight ______ Date/Time ________

Stretch ◯   Warm-Up ________________________________

Strength Training

Exercise		Set 1	Set 2	Set 3	Set 4	Set 5	Set 6
	Reps						
	Weight						
	Reps						
	Weight						
	Reps						
	Weight						
	Reps						
	Weight						
	Reps						
	Weight						
	Reps						
	Weight						
	Reps						
	Weight						
	Reps						
	Weight						
	Reps						
	Weight						
	Reps						
	Weight						

Cardio

Exercise	Calories	Distance	Time

Water Intake ________________

Cooldown ________________

Feeling ☆ ☆ ☆ ☆ ☆

Notes

Today's Goal

Today's Goal __________________________   (M) (T) (W) (T) (F) (S) (S)

Muscle Group Focus __________________________   Weight ________   Date/Time ________

Stretch ◯   Warm-Up __________________________

Strength Training

Exercise		Set 1	Set 2	Set 3	Set 4	Set 5	Set 6
	Reps						
	Weight						
	Reps						
	Weight						
	Reps						
	Weight						
	Reps						
	Weight						
	Reps						
	Weight						
	Reps						
	Weight						
	Reps						
	Weight						
	Reps						
	Weight						
	Reps						
	Weight						
	Reps						
	Weight						

Cardio

Exercise	Calories	Distance	Time

Water Intake __________________________

Cooldown __________________________

Feeling ☆ ☆ ☆ ☆ ☆

Notes

Today's Goal

Muscle Group Focus ____________________ Weight ______ Date/Time ________

Stretch ◯   Warm-Up ____________________________________

Strength Training

Exercise		Set 1	Set 2	Set 3	Set 4	Set 5	Set 6
	Reps						
	Weight						
	Reps						
	Weight						
	Reps						
	Weight						
	Reps						
	Weight						
	Reps						
	Weight						
	Reps						
	Weight						
	Reps						
	Weight						
	Reps						
	Weight						
	Reps						
	Weight						
	Reps						
	Weight						

Cardio

Exercise	Calories	Distance	Time

Water Intake ________________

Cooldown ________________

Feeling ☆ ☆ ☆ ☆ ☆

Notes

Today's Goal

M T W T F **S** **S**

Muscle Group Focus ______________________ Weight ______ Date/Time ______

Stretch ○   Warm-Up ______________________

Strength Training

Exercise		Set 1	Set 2	Set 3	Set 4	Set 5	Set 6
	Reps						
	Weight						
	Reps						
	Weight						
	Reps						
	Weight						
	Reps						
	Weight						
	Reps						
	Weight						
	Reps						
	Weight						
	Reps						
	Weight						
	Reps						
	Weight						
	Reps						
	Weight						
	Reps						
	Weight						

Cardio

Exercise	Calories	Distance	Time

Water Intake ______

Cooldown ______

Feeling ☆ ☆ ☆ ☆ ☆

Notes

Today's Goal

M T W T F **S** **S**

Muscle Group Focus ___________________________ Weight _______ Date/Time _______

Stretch ◯   Warm-Up ___________________________________

Strength Training

Exercise		Set 1	Set 2	Set 3	Set 4	Set 5	Set 6
	Reps						
	Weight						
	Reps						
	Weight						
	Reps						
	Weight						
	Reps						
	Weight						
	Reps						
	Weight						
	Reps						
	Weight						
	Reps						
	Weight						
	Reps						
	Weight						
	Reps						
	Weight						
	Reps						
	Weight						

Cardio

Exercise	Calories	Distance	Time

Water Intake ___________

Cooldown ___________

Feeling ☆ ☆ ☆ ☆ ☆

Notes

Today's Goal

M T W T F **S** **S**

Muscle Group Focus ___________________ Weight _______ Date/Time _______

Stretch ◯   Warm-Up ___________________________________

Strength Training

Exercise		Set 1	Set 2	Set 3	Set 4	Set 5	Set 6
	Reps						
	Weight						
	Reps						
	Weight						
	Reps						
	Weight						
	Reps						
	Weight						
	Reps						
	Weight						
	Reps						
	Weight						
	Reps						
	Weight						
	Reps						
	Weight						
	Reps						
	Weight						

Cardio

Exercise	Calories	Distance	Time

Water Intake ___________________

Cooldown ___________________

Feeling ☆ ☆ ☆ ☆ ☆

Notes

Today's Goal

(M) (T) (W) (T) (F) (S) (S)

Muscle Group Focus ___________________ Weight _______ Date/Time _______

Stretch ◯   Warm-Up _______________________________

Strength Training

Exercise		Set 1	Set 2	Set 3	Set 4	Set 5	Set 6
	Reps						
	Weight						
	Reps						
	Weight						
	Reps						
	Weight						
	Reps						
	Weight						
	Reps						
	Weight						
	Reps						
	Weight						
	Reps						
	Weight						
	Reps						
	Weight						
	Reps						
	Weight						

Cardio

Exercise	Calories	Distance	Time

Water Intake _______________

Cooldown _______________

Feeling ☆ ☆ ☆ ☆ ☆

Notes

Today's Goal

M T W T F **S** **S**

Muscle Group Focus ___________________ Weight _______ Date/Time _______

Stretch ◯   Warm-Up ___________________

Strength Training

Exercise		Set 1	Set 2	Set 3	Set 4	Set 5	Set 6
	Reps						
	Weight						
	Reps						
	Weight						
	Reps						
	Weight						
	Reps						
	Weight						
	Reps						
	Weight						
	Reps						
	Weight						
	Reps						
	Weight						
	Reps						
	Weight						
	Reps						
	Weight						
	Reps						
	Weight						

Cardio

Exercise	Calories	Distance	Time

Water Intake ___________

Cooldown ___________

Feeling ☆ ☆ ☆ ☆ ☆

Notes

Today's Goal

M T W T F **S** **S**

Muscle Group Focus ____________________ Weight ______ Date/Time ______

Stretch ◯   Warm-Up ________________________

Strength Training

Exercise		Set 1	Set 2	Set 3	Set 4	Set 5	Set 6
	Reps						
	Weight						
	Reps						
	Weight						
	Reps						
	Weight						
	Reps						
	Weight						
	Reps						
	Weight						
	Reps						
	Weight						
	Reps						
	Weight						
	Reps						
	Weight						

Cardio

Exercise	Calories	Distance	Time

Water Intake ________________

Cooldown ________________

Feeling ☆ ☆ ☆ ☆ ☆

Notes

Today's Goal

Today's Goal ___________________ M T W T F **S** **S**

Muscle Group Focus ___________________ Weight _______ Date/Time _______

Stretch ◯ Warm-Up ___________________

Strength Training

Exercise		Set 1	Set 2	Set 3	Set 4	Set 5	Set 6
	Reps						
	Weight						
	Reps						
	Weight						
	Reps						
	Weight						
	Reps						
	Weight						
	Reps						
	Weight						
	Reps						
	Weight						
	Reps						
	Weight						
	Reps						
	Weight						
	Reps						
	Weight						

Cardio

Exercise	Calories	Distance	Time

Water Intake ___________________

Cooldown ___________________

Feeling ☆ ☆ ☆ ☆ ☆

Notes

Today's Goal

M T W T F S S

Muscle Group Focus ____________________ Weight ________ Date/Time ________

Stretch ◯   Warm-Up ____________________

Strength Training

Exercise		Set 1	Set 2	Set 3	Set 4	Set 5	Set 6
	Reps						
	Weight						
	Reps						
	Weight						
	Reps						
	Weight						
	Reps						
	Weight						
	Reps						
	Weight						
	Reps						
	Weight						
	Reps						
	Weight						
	Reps						
	Weight						
	Reps						
	Weight						

Cardio

Exercise	Calories	Distance	Time

Water Intake ____________________

Cooldown ____________________

Feeling ☆ ☆ ☆ ☆ ☆

Notes

Today's Goal

  M   T   W   T   F   **S**   **S**

Muscle Group Focus   Weight   Date/Time

Stretch ◯   Warm-Up

Strength Training

Exercise		Set 1	Set 2	Set 3	Set 4	Set 5	Set 6
	Reps						
	Weight						
	Reps						
	Weight						
	Reps						
	Weight						
	Reps						
	Weight						
	Reps						
	Weight						
	Reps						
	Weight						
	Reps						
	Weight						
	Reps						
	Weight						
	Reps						
	Weight						
	Reps						
	Weight						

Cardio

Exercise	Calories	Distance	Time

Water Intake

Cooldown

Feeling ☆ ☆ ☆ ☆ ☆

Notes

Today's Goal

M T W T F S S

Muscle Group Focus ___________________ Weight _______ Date/Time _______

Stretch ◯   Warm-Up ___________________

Strength Training

Exercise		Set 1	Set 2	Set 3	Set 4	Set 5	Set 6
	Reps						
	Weight						
	Reps						
	Weight						
	Reps						
	Weight						
	Reps						
	Weight						
	Reps						
	Weight						
	Reps						
	Weight						
	Reps						
	Weight						
	Reps						
	Weight						
	Reps						
	Weight						

Cardio

Exercise	Calories	Distance	Time

Water Intake ___________________

Cooldown ___________________

Feeling ☆ ☆ ☆ ☆ ☆

Notes

Today's Goal

(M) (T) (W) (T) (F) (**S**) (**S**)

Muscle Group Focus ________________________ Weight ________ Date/Time __________

Stretch ◯   Warm-Up ____

Strength Training

Exercise		Set 1	Set 2	Set 3	Set 4	Set 5	Set 6
	Reps						
	Weight						
	Reps						
	Weight						
	Reps						
	Weight						
	Reps						
	Weight						
	Reps						
	Weight						
	Reps						
	Weight						
	Reps						
	Weight						
	Reps						
	Weight						
	Reps						
	Weight						
	Reps						
	Weight						

Cardio

Exercise	Calories	Distance	Time

Water Intake __________

Cooldown __________

Feeling ☆ ☆ ☆ ☆ ☆

Notes

Today's Goal   __________________________ Ⓜ Ⓣ Ⓦ Ⓣ Ⓕ Ⓢ Ⓢ

Muscle Group Focus __________________________ Weight ________ Date/Time ________

Stretch ◯   Warm-Up __________________________

Strength Training

Exercise		Set 1	Set 2	Set 3	Set 4	Set 5	Set 6
	Reps						
	Weight						
	Reps						
	Weight						
	Reps						
	Weight						
	Reps						
	Weight						
	Reps						
	Weight						
	Reps						
	Weight						
	Reps						
	Weight						
	Reps						
	Weight						
	Reps						
	Weight						
	Reps						
	Weight						

Cardio

Exercise	Calories	Distance	Time

Water Intake __________________________

Cooldown __________________________

Feeling ☆ ☆ ☆ ☆ ☆

Notes

Today's Goal

Muscle Group Focus

Weight _______   Date/Time _______

Stretch ◯   Warm-Up

Strength Training

Exercise		Set 1	Set 2	Set 3	Set 4	Set 5	Set 6
	Reps						
	Weight						
	Reps						
	Weight						
	Reps						
	Weight						
	Reps						
	Weight						
	Reps						
	Weight						
	Reps						
	Weight						
	Reps						
	Weight						
	Reps						
	Weight						
	Reps						
	Weight						

Cardio

Exercise	Calories	Distance	Time

Water Intake

Cooldown

Feeling ☆ ☆ ☆ ☆ ☆

Notes

Today's Goal

_______________________   Ⓜ Ⓣ Ⓦ Ⓣ Ⓕ Ⓢ Ⓢ

Muscle Group Focus _______________   Weight ______   Date/Time ______

Stretch ◯   Warm-Up _______________________

Strength Training

Exercise		Set 1	Set 2	Set 3	Set 4	Set 5	Set 6
	Reps						
	Weight						
	Reps						
	Weight						
	Reps						
	Weight						
	Reps						
	Weight						
	Reps						
	Weight						
	Reps						
	Weight						
	Reps						
	Weight						
	Reps						
	Weight						
	Reps						
	Weight						
	Reps						
	Weight						

Cardio

Exercise	Calories	Distance	Time

Water Intake _______________

Cooldown _______________

Feeling ☆ ☆ ☆ ☆ ☆

Notes

Today's Goal

M T W T F **S** **S**

Muscle Group Focus ________________ Weight ________ Date/Time ________

Stretch ◯   Warm-Up ________________

Strength Training

Exercise		Set 1	Set 2	Set 3	Set 4	Set 5	Set 6
	Reps						
	Weight						
	Reps						
	Weight						
	Reps						
	Weight						
	Reps						
	Weight						
	Reps						
	Weight						
	Reps						
	Weight						
	Reps						
	Weight						
	Reps						
	Weight						
	Reps						
	Weight						
	Reps						
	Weight						

Cardio

Exercise	Calories	Distance	Time

Water Intake ________________

Cooldown ________________

Feeling ☆ ☆ ☆ ☆ ☆

Notes

Today's Goal

(M) (T) (W) (T) (F) (S) (S)

Muscle Group Focus   Weight   Date/Time

Stretch ◯   Warm-Up

Strength Training

Exercise		Set 1	Set 2	Set 3	Set 4	Set 5	Set 6
	Reps						
	Weight						
	Reps						
	Weight						
	Reps						
	Weight						
	Reps						
	Weight						
	Reps						
	Weight						
	Reps						
	Weight						
	Reps						
	Weight						
	Reps						
	Weight						
	Reps						
	Weight						
	Reps						
	Weight						

Cardio

Exercise	Calories	Distance	Time

Water Intake

Cooldown

Feeling ☆ ☆ ☆ ☆ ☆

Notes

Today's Goal

_________________________________   Ⓜ Ⓣ Ⓦ Ⓣ Ⓕ ⬤S ⬤S

Muscle Group Focus _____________________   Weight _______   Date/Time _________

Stretch ◯   Warm-Up _______________________________________

Strength Training

Exercise		Set 1	Set 2	Set 3	Set 4	Set 5	Set 6
	Reps						
	Weight						
	Reps						
	Weight						
	Reps						
	Weight						
	Reps						
	Weight						
	Reps						
	Weight						
	Reps						
	Weight						
	Reps						
	Weight						
	Reps						
	Weight						
	Reps						
	Weight						

Cardio

Exercise	Calories	Distance	Time

Water Intake _____________

Cooldown _____________

Feeling ☆ ☆ ☆ ☆ ☆

Notes

Today's Goal

M T W T F **S** **S**

Muscle Group Focus __________________________ Weight ________ Date/Time ________

Stretch ◯   Warm-Up ____________________________________

Strength Training

Exercise		Set 1	Set 2	Set 3	Set 4	Set 5	Set 6
	Reps						
	Weight						
	Reps						
	Weight						
	Reps						
	Weight						
	Reps						
	Weight						
	Reps						
	Weight						
	Reps						
	Weight						
	Reps						
	Weight						
	Reps						
	Weight						
	Reps						
	Weight						
	Reps						
	Weight						

Cardio

Exercise	Calories	Distance	Time

Water Intake ____________________

Cooldown ____________________

Feeling ☆ ☆ ☆ ☆ ☆

Notes

Today's Goal

M T W T F S S

Muscle Group Focus ________________ Weight ________ Date/Time ________

Stretch ◯   Warm-Up ________________________________

Strength Training

Exercise		Set 1	Set 2	Set 3	Set 4	Set 5	Set 6
	Reps						
	Weight						
	Reps						
	Weight						
	Reps						
	Weight						
	Reps						
	Weight						
	Reps						
	Weight						
	Reps						
	Weight						
	Reps						
	Weight						
	Reps						
	Weight						

Cardio

Exercise	Calories	Distance	Time

Water Intake ________________

Cooldown ________________

Feeling ☆ ☆ ☆ ☆ ☆

Notes

Today's Goal

M T W T F **S** **S**

Muscle Group Focus ___________________ Weight _______ Date/Time _______

Stretch ◯   Warm-Up _______________________________

Strength Training

Exercise		Set 1	Set 2	Set 3	Set 4	Set 5	Set 6
	Reps						
	Weight						
	Reps						
	Weight						
	Reps						
	Weight						
	Reps						
	Weight						
	Reps						
	Weight						
	Reps						
	Weight						
	Reps						
	Weight						
	Reps						
	Weight						
	Reps						
	Weight						
	Reps						
	Weight						

Cardio

Exercise	Calories	Distance	Time

Water Intake _______________

Cooldown _______________

Feeling ☆ ☆ ☆ ☆ ☆

Notes

Today's Goal

M T W T F **S** **S**

Muscle Group Focus ____________________ Weight ________ Date/Time __________

Stretch ◯ Warm-Up ____

Strength Training

Exercise		Set 1	Set 2	Set 3	Set 4	Set 5	Set 6
	Reps						
	Weight						
	Reps						
	Weight						
	Reps						
	Weight						
	Reps						
	Weight						
	Reps						
	Weight						
	Reps						
	Weight						
	Reps						
	Weight						
	Reps						
	Weight						
	Reps						
	Weight						
	Reps						
	Weight						

Cardio

Exercise	Calories	Distance	Time

Water Intake __________

Cooldown __________

Feeling ☆ ☆ ☆ ☆ ☆

Notes

Today's Goal

(M) (T) (W) (T) (F) (S) (S)

Muscle Group Focus ________________________ Weight ________ Date/Time ________

Stretch ◯   Warm-Up ________________________________

Strength Training

Exercise		Set 1	Set 2	Set 3	Set 4	Set 5	Set 6
	Reps						
	Weight						
	Reps						
	Weight						
	Reps						
	Weight						
	Reps						
	Weight						
	Reps						
	Weight						
	Reps						
	Weight						
	Reps						
	Weight						
	Reps						
	Weight						
	Reps						
	Weight						

Cardio

Exercise	Calories	Distance	Time

Water Intake ________________

Cooldown ________________

Feeling ☆ ☆ ☆ ☆ ☆

Notes

Today's Goal

M T W T F S S

Muscle Group Focus ______________________ Weight ________ Date/Time __________

Stretch ◯   Warm-Up ______________________

Strength Training

Exercise		Set 1	Set 2	Set 3	Set 4	Set 5	Set 6
	Reps						
	Weight						
	Reps						
	Weight						
	Reps						
	Weight						
	Reps						
	Weight						
	Reps						
	Weight						
	Reps						
	Weight						
	Reps						
	Weight						
	Reps						
	Weight						
	Reps						
	Weight						

Cardio

Exercise	Calories	Distance	Time

Water Intake ______________________

Cooldown ______________________

Feeling ☆ ☆ ☆ ☆ ☆

Notes

Today's Goal

(M) (T) (W) (T) (F) **(S)** **(S)**

Muscle Group Focus ___________________ Weight _______ Date/Time _______

Stretch ◯   Warm-Up ___________________

Strength Training

Exercise		Set 1	Set 2	Set 3	Set 4	Set 5	Set 6
	Reps						
	Weight						
	Reps						
	Weight						
	Reps						
	Weight						
	Reps						
	Weight						
	Reps						
	Weight						
	Reps						
	Weight						
	Reps						
	Weight						
	Reps						
	Weight						
	Reps						
	Weight						
	Reps						
	Weight						

Cardio

Exercise	Calories	Distance	Time

Water Intake ___________________

Cooldown ___________________

Feeling ☆ ☆ ☆ ☆ ☆

Notes

Today's Goal

Today's Goal ___________________ M T W T F **S** **S**

Muscle Group Focus ___________________ Weight _______ Date/Time _______

Stretch ◯ Warm-Up ___________________

Strength Training

Exercise		Set 1	Set 2	Set 3	Set 4	Set 5	Set 6
	Reps						
	Weight						
	Reps						
	Weight						
	Reps						
	Weight						
	Reps						
	Weight						
	Reps						
	Weight						
	Reps						
	Weight						
	Reps						
	Weight						
	Reps						
	Weight						
	Reps						
	Weight						
	Reps						
	Weight						

Cardio

Exercise	Calories	Distance	Time

Water Intake ___________________

Cooldown ___________________

Feeling ☆ ☆ ☆ ☆ ☆

Notes

Today's Goal

M T W T F S S

Muscle Group Focus ___________________________ Weight _______ Date/Time _______

Stretch ◯   Warm-Up _______________________________

Strength Training

Exercise		Set 1	Set 2	Set 3	Set 4	Set 5	Set 6
	Reps						
	Weight						
	Reps						
	Weight						
	Reps						
	Weight						
	Reps						
	Weight						
	Reps						
	Weight						
	Reps						
	Weight						
	Reps						
	Weight						
	Reps						
	Weight						
	Reps						
	Weight						

Cardio

Exercise	Calories	Distance	Time

Water Intake _______________

Cooldown _______________

Feeling ☆ ☆ ☆ ☆ ☆

Notes

Today's Goal

M T W T F **S** **S**

Muscle Group Focus ______________________ Weight ______ Date/Time ______

Stretch ◯   Warm-Up ______________________

Strength Training

Exercise		Set 1	Set 2	Set 3	Set 4	Set 5	Set 6
	Reps						
	Weight						
	Reps						
	Weight						
	Reps						
	Weight						
	Reps						
	Weight						
	Reps						
	Weight						
	Reps						
	Weight						
	Reps						
	Weight						
	Reps						
	Weight						
	Reps						
	Weight						
	Reps						
	Weight						

Cardio

Exercise	Calories	Distance	Time

Water Intake ______________________

Cooldown ______________________

Feeling ☆ ☆ ☆ ☆ ☆

Notes

Today's Goal

M T W **T** F **S** **S**

Muscle Group Focus ______________________ Weight ______ Date/Time ______

Stretch ○ Warm-Up ______________________

Strength Training

Exercise		Set 1	Set 2	Set 3	Set 4	Set 5	Set 6
	Reps						
	Weight						
	Reps						
	Weight						
	Reps						
	Weight						
	Reps						
	Weight						
	Reps						
	Weight						
	Reps						
	Weight						
	Reps						
	Weight						
	Reps						
	Weight						
	Reps						
	Weight						

Cardio

Exercise	Calories	Distance	Time

Water Intake ______________________

Cooldown ______________________

Feeling ☆ ☆ ☆ ☆ ☆

Notes

Today's Goal

(M) (T) (W) (T) (F) (S) (S)

Muscle Group Focus _______________________ Weight _______ Date/Time _______

Stretch ○   Warm-Up _______________________

Strength Training

Exercise		Set 1	Set 2	Set 3	Set 4	Set 5	Set 6
	Reps						
	Weight						
	Reps						
	Weight						
	Reps						
	Weight						
	Reps						
	Weight						
	Reps						
	Weight						
	Reps						
	Weight						
	Reps						
	Weight						
	Reps						
	Weight						
	Reps						
	Weight						

Cardio

Exercise	Calories	Distance	Time

Water Intake _______________________

Cooldown _______________________

Feeling ☆ ☆ ☆ ☆ ☆

Notes

Today's Goal

M T W T F **S** **S**

Muscle Group Focus __________ Weight ______ Date/Time ______

Stretch ○   Warm-Up __________

Strength Training

Exercise		Set 1	Set 2	Set 3	Set 4	Set 5	Set 6
	Reps						
	Weight						
	Reps						
	Weight						
	Reps						
	Weight						
	Reps						
	Weight						
	Reps						
	Weight						
	Reps						
	Weight						
	Reps						
	Weight						
	Reps						
	Weight						
	Reps						
	Weight						

Cardio

Exercise	Calories	Distance	Time

Water Intake __________

Cooldown __________

Feeling ☆ ☆ ☆ ☆ ☆

Notes

Today's Goal

_______________________________ Ⓜ Ⓣ Ⓦ Ⓣ Ⓕ ⬤S ⬤S

Muscle Group Focus _______________________ Weight _______ Date/Time _______

Stretch ○   Warm-Up _______________________________________

Strength Training

Exercise		Set 1	Set 2	Set 3	Set 4	Set 5	Set 6
	Reps						
	Weight						
	Reps						
	Weight						
	Reps						
	Weight						
	Reps						
	Weight						
	Reps						
	Weight						
	Reps						
	Weight						
	Reps						
	Weight						
	Reps						
	Weight						
	Reps						
	Weight						

Cardio

Exercise	Calories	Distance	Time

Water Intake _______________

Cooldown _______________

Feeling ☆ ☆ ☆ ☆ ☆

Notes

Today's Goal

M T W T F **S** **S**

Muscle Group Focus ______________________ Weight ______ Date/Time ______

Stretch ○   Warm-Up ______________________

Strength Training

Exercise		Set 1	Set 2	Set 3	Set 4	Set 5	Set 6
	Reps						
	Weight						
	Reps						
	Weight						
	Reps						
	Weight						
	Reps						
	Weight						
	Reps						
	Weight						
	Reps						
	Weight						
	Reps						
	Weight						
	Reps						
	Weight						
	Reps						
	Weight						

Cardio

Exercise	Calories	Distance	Time

Water Intake ______________________

Cooldown ______________________

Feeling ☆ ☆ ☆ ☆ ☆

Notes

Today's Goal

(M) (T) (W) (T) (F) (**S**) (**S**)

Muscle Group Focus ____________________ Weight _______ Date/Time _______

Stretch ◯   Warm-Up ____________________

Strength Training

Exercise		Set 1	Set 2	Set 3	Set 4	Set 5	Set 6
	Reps						
	Weight						
	Reps						
	Weight						
	Reps						
	Weight						
	Reps						
	Weight						
	Reps						
	Weight						
	Reps						
	Weight						
	Reps						
	Weight						
	Reps						
	Weight						
	Reps						
	Weight						

Cardio

Exercise	Calories	Distance	Time

Water Intake ____________________

Cooldown ____________________

Feeling ☆ ☆ ☆ ☆ ☆

Notes

Today's Goal _______________________

(M) (T) (W) (T) (F) (S) (S)

Muscle Group Focus _______________________ Weight _______ Date/Time _______

Stretch ◯   Warm-Up _______________________

Strength Training

Exercise		Set 1	Set 2	Set 3	Set 4	Set 5	Set 6
	Reps						
	Weight						
	Reps						
	Weight						
	Reps						
	Weight						
	Reps						
	Weight						
	Reps						
	Weight						
	Reps						
	Weight						
	Reps						
	Weight						
	Reps						
	Weight						
	Reps						
	Weight						

Cardio

Exercise	Calories	Distance	Time

Water Intake _______________________

Cooldown _______________________

Feeling ☆ ☆ ☆ ☆ ☆

Notes

Today's Goal

M T W T F **S** **S**

Muscle Group Focus _______________ Weight _______ Date/Time _______

Stretch ◯   Warm-Up _______________

Strength Training

Exercise		Set 1	Set 2	Set 3	Set 4	Set 5	Set 6
	Reps						
	Weight						
	Reps						
	Weight						
	Reps						
	Weight						
	Reps						
	Weight						
	Reps						
	Weight						
	Reps						
	Weight						
	Reps						
	Weight						
	Reps						
	Weight						
	Reps						
	Weight						
	Reps						
	Weight						

Cardio

Exercise	Calories	Distance	Time

Water Intake _______________

Cooldown _______________

Feeling ☆ ☆ ☆ ☆ ☆

Notes

Today's Goal

M T W T F **S** **S**

Muscle Group Focus ________________ Weight ________ Date/Time ________

Stretch ◯   Warm-Up ________________

Strength Training

Exercise		Set 1	Set 2	Set 3	Set 4	Set 5	Set 6
	Reps						
	Weight						
	Reps						
	Weight						
	Reps						
	Weight						
	Reps						
	Weight						
	Reps						
	Weight						
	Reps						
	Weight						
	Reps						
	Weight						
	Reps						
	Weight						
	Reps						
	Weight						
	Reps						
	Weight						

Cardio

Exercise	Calories	Distance	Time

Water Intake ________________

Cooldown ________________

Feeling ☆ ☆ ☆ ☆ ☆

Notes

Today's Goal

M T W T F **S** **S**

Muscle Group Focus ___________________ Weight ________ Date/Time ________

Stretch ◯ Warm-Up ___________________

Strength Training

Exercise		Set 1	Set 2	Set 3	Set 4	Set 5	Set 6
	Reps						
	Weight						
	Reps						
	Weight						
	Reps						
	Weight						
	Reps						
	Weight						
	Reps						
	Weight						
	Reps						
	Weight						
	Reps						
	Weight						
	Reps						
	Weight						
	Reps						
	Weight						

Cardio

Exercise	Calories	Distance	Time

Water Intake ___________________

Cooldown ___________________

Feeling ☆ ☆ ☆ ☆ ☆

Notes

Today's Goal

(M) (T) (W) (T) (F) (**S**) (**S**)

Muscle Group Focus ___________________ Weight _______ Date/Time _______

Stretch ○   Warm-Up ___________________

Strength Training

Exercise		Set 1	Set 2	Set 3	Set 4	Set 5	Set 6
	Reps						
	Weight						
	Reps						
	Weight						
	Reps						
	Weight						
	Reps						
	Weight						
	Reps						
	Weight						
	Reps						
	Weight						
	Reps						
	Weight						
	Reps						
	Weight						
	Reps						
	Weight						
	Reps						
	Weight						

Cardio

Exercise	Calories	Distance	Time

Water Intake ___________________

Cooldown ___________________

Feeling ☆ ☆ ☆ ☆ ☆

Notes

Today's Goal

(M) (T) (W) (T) (F) (**S**) (**S**)

Muscle Group Focus ________________________ Weight ________ Date/Time ________

Stretch ○   Warm-Up ________________________

Strength Training

Exercise		Set 1	Set 2	Set 3	Set 4	Set 5	Set 6
	Reps						
	Weight						
	Reps						
	Weight						
	Reps						
	Weight						
	Reps						
	Weight						
	Reps						
	Weight						
	Reps						
	Weight						
	Reps						
	Weight						
	Reps						
	Weight						
	Reps						
	Weight						
	Reps						
	Weight						

Cardio

Exercise	Calories	Distance	Time

Water Intake ________________

Cooldown ________________

Feeling ☆ ☆ ☆ ☆ ☆

Notes

Today's Goal _______________________   M T W T F **S** **S**

Muscle Group Focus _________________________   Weight _______   Date/Time _______

Stretch ◯   Warm-Up _______________________________

Strength Training

Exercise		Set 1	Set 2	Set 3	Set 4	Set 5	Set 6
	Reps						
	Weight						
	Reps						
	Weight						
	Reps						
	Weight						
	Reps						
	Weight						
	Reps						
	Weight						
	Reps						
	Weight						
	Reps						
	Weight						
	Reps						
	Weight						
	Reps						
	Weight						
	Reps						
	Weight						

Cardio

Exercise	Calories	Distance	Time

Water Intake _______________

Cooldown _______________

Feeling ☆ ☆ ☆ ☆ ☆

Notes

Today's Goal

M T W T F **S** **S**

Muscle Group Focus ______________________ Weight ________ Date/Time __________

Stretch ◯   Warm-Up ______________________

Strength Training

Exercise		Set 1	Set 2	Set 3	Set 4	Set 5	Set 6
	Reps						
	Weight						
	Reps						
	Weight						
	Reps						
	Weight						
	Reps						
	Weight						
	Reps						
	Weight						
	Reps						
	Weight						
	Reps						
	Weight						
	Reps						
	Weight						
	Reps						
	Weight						
	Reps						
	Weight						

Cardio

Exercise	Calories	Distance	Time

Water Intake ______________________

Cooldown ______________________

Feeling ☆ ☆ ☆ ☆ ☆

Notes

Today's Goal

M T W T F **S** **S**

Muscle Group Focus ____________________ Weight ________ Date/Time ________

Stretch ◯ Warm-Up ____________________

Strength Training

Exercise		Set 1	Set 2	Set 3	Set 4	Set 5	Set 6
	Reps						
	Weight						
	Reps						
	Weight						
	Reps						
	Weight						
	Reps						
	Weight						
	Reps						
	Weight						
	Reps						
	Weight						
	Reps						
	Weight						
	Reps						
	Weight						
	Reps						
	Weight						

Cardio

Exercise	Calories	Distance	Time

Water Intake ____________________

Cooldown ____________________

Feeling ☆ ☆ ☆ ☆ ☆

Notes

Today's Goal

M T W T F **S** **S**

Muscle Group Focus ______________ Weight ______ Date/Time ______

Stretch ◯ Warm-Up ______________

Strength Training

Exercise		Set 1	Set 2	Set 3	Set 4	Set 5	Set 6
	Reps						
	Weight						
	Reps						
	Weight						
	Reps						
	Weight						
	Reps						
	Weight						
	Reps						
	Weight						
	Reps						
	Weight						
	Reps						
	Weight						
	Reps						
	Weight						
	Reps						
	Weight						
	Reps						
	Weight						

Cardio

Exercise	Calories	Distance	Time

Water Intake ______________

Cooldown ______________

Feeling ☆ ☆ ☆ ☆ ☆

Notes

Today's Goal

(M) (T) (W) (T) (F) (S) (S)

Muscle Group Focus ____________________ Weight _______ Date/Time _______

Stretch ◯   Warm-Up ___________________________________

Strength Training

Exercise		Set 1	Set 2	Set 3	Set 4	Set 5	Set 6
	Reps						
	Weight						
	Reps						
	Weight						
	Reps						
	Weight						
	Reps						
	Weight						
	Reps						
	Weight						
	Reps						
	Weight						
	Reps						
	Weight						
	Reps						
	Weight						
	Reps						
	Weight						
	Reps						
	Weight						

Cardio

Exercise	Calories	Distance	Time

Water Intake ___________________

Cooldown ___________________

Feeling ☆ ☆ ☆ ☆ ☆

Notes

Today's Goal ______________________ Ⓜ Ⓣ Ⓦ Ⓣ Ⓕ ⬤S ⬤S

Muscle Group Focus ________________   Weight ______   Date/Time ______

Stretch ◯   Warm-Up ______________________

Strength Training

Exercise		Set 1	Set 2	Set 3	Set 4	Set 5	Set 6
	Reps						
	Weight						
	Reps						
	Weight						
	Reps						
	Weight						
	Reps						
	Weight						
	Reps						
	Weight						
	Reps						
	Weight						
	Reps						
	Weight						
	Reps						
	Weight						
	Reps						
	Weight						

Cardio

Exercise	Calories	Distance	Time

Water Intake ______________

Cooldown ______________

Feeling ☆ ☆ ☆ ☆ ☆

Notes

Today's Goal

M T W T F **S** **S**

Muscle Group Focus __________________ Weight ________ Date/Time ________

Stretch ◯   Warm-Up ________________________

Strength Training

Exercise		Set 1	Set 2	Set 3	Set 4	Set 5	Set 6
	Reps						
	Weight						
	Reps						
	Weight						
	Reps						
	Weight						
	Reps						
	Weight						
	Reps						
	Weight						
	Reps						
	Weight						
	Reps						
	Weight						
	Reps						
	Weight						
	Reps						
	Weight						
	Reps						
	Weight						

Cardio

Exercise	Calories	Distance	Time

Water Intake ________

Cooldown ________

Feeling ☆ ☆ ☆ ☆ ☆

Notes

Today's Goal

(M) (T) (W) (T) (F) **(S) (S)**

Muscle Group Focus _______________ Weight ______ Date/Time ______

Stretch ◯   Warm-Up _______________

Strength Training

Exercise		Set 1	Set 2	Set 3	Set 4	Set 5	Set 6
	Reps						
	Weight						
	Reps						
	Weight						
	Reps						
	Weight						
	Reps						
	Weight						
	Reps						
	Weight						
	Reps						
	Weight						
	Reps						
	Weight						
	Reps						
	Weight						
	Reps						
	Weight						

Cardio

Exercise	Calories	Distance	Time

Water Intake _______________

Cooldown _______________

Feeling ☆ ☆ ☆ ☆ ☆

Notes

Today's Goal _______________________ Ⓜ Ⓣ Ⓦ Ⓣ Ⓕ ⬤S ⬤S

Muscle Group Focus _______________________   Weight _______   Date/Time _______

Stretch ◯   Warm-Up _______________________

Strength Training

Exercise		Set 1	Set 2	Set 3	Set 4	Set 5	Set 6
	Reps						
	Weight						
	Reps						
	Weight						
	Reps						
	Weight						
	Reps						
	Weight						
	Reps						
	Weight						
	Reps						
	Weight						
	Reps						
	Weight						
	Reps						
	Weight						
	Reps						
	Weight						
	Reps						
	Weight						

Cardio

Exercise	Calories	Distance	Time

Water Intake _______________________

Cooldown _______________________

Feeling ☆ ☆ ☆ ☆ ☆

Notes

Today's Goal

(M) (T) (W) (T) (F) **(S)** **(S)**

Muscle Group Focus ___________________ Weight _______ Date/Time _______

Stretch ◯   Warm-Up _______________________________

Strength Training

Exercise		Set 1	Set 2	Set 3	Set 4	Set 5	Set 6
	Reps						
	Weight						
	Reps						
	Weight						
	Reps						
	Weight						
	Reps						
	Weight						
	Reps						
	Weight						
	Reps						
	Weight						
	Reps						
	Weight						
	Reps						
	Weight						
	Reps						
	Weight						

Cardio

Exercise	Calories	Distance	Time

Water Intake _______

Cooldown _______

Feeling ☆ ☆ ☆ ☆ ☆

Notes

Today's Goal

M (T) (W) (T) (F) **S** **S**

Muscle Group Focus _______________ Weight _______ Date/Time _______

Stretch ◯   Warm-Up _______________________

Strength Training

Exercise		Set 1	Set 2	Set 3	Set 4	Set 5	Set 6
	Reps						
	Weight						
	Reps						
	Weight						
	Reps						
	Weight						
	Reps						
	Weight						
	Reps						
	Weight						
	Reps						
	Weight						
	Reps						
	Weight						
	Reps						
	Weight						
	Reps						
	Weight						

Cardio

Exercise	Calories	Distance	Time

Water Intake _______________

Cooldown _______________

Feeling ☆ ☆ ☆ ☆ ☆

Notes

Today's Goal

M T W T F **S** **S**

Muscle Group Focus ____________________   Weight ________   Date/Time __________

Stretch ◯   Warm-Up ____________________

Strength Training

Exercise		Set 1	Set 2	Set 3	Set 4	Set 5	Set 6
	Reps						
	Weight						
	Reps						
	Weight						
	Reps						
	Weight						
	Reps						
	Weight						
	Reps						
	Weight						
	Reps						
	Weight						
	Reps						
	Weight						
	Reps						
	Weight						
	Reps						
	Weight						
	Reps						
	Weight						

Cardio

Exercise	Calories	Distance	Time

Water Intake ____________________

Cooldown ____________________

Feeling ☆ ☆ ☆ ☆ ☆

Notes

Today's Goal

M T W T F S S

Muscle Group Focus _______________________ Weight _______ Date/Time _______

Stretch ◯   Warm-Up _______________________

Strength Training

Exercise		Set 1	Set 2	Set 3	Set 4	Set 5	Set 6
	Reps						
	Weight						
	Reps						
	Weight						
	Reps						
	Weight						
	Reps						
	Weight						
	Reps						
	Weight						
	Reps						
	Weight						
	Reps						
	Weight						
	Reps						
	Weight						
	Reps						
	Weight						

Cardio

Exercise	Calories	Distance	Time

Water Intake _______________________

Cooldown _______________________

Feeling ☆ ☆ ☆ ☆ ☆

Notes

Today's Goal

M T W T F **S** **S**

Muscle Group Focus ______________________ Weight ________ Date/Time __________

Stretch ◯   Warm-Up ______________________

Strength Training

Exercise		Set 1	Set 2	Set 3	Set 4	Set 5	Set 6
	Reps						
	Weight						
	Reps						
	Weight						
	Reps						
	Weight						
	Reps						
	Weight						
	Reps						
	Weight						
	Reps						
	Weight						
	Reps						
	Weight						
	Reps						
	Weight						
	Reps						
	Weight						

Cardio

Exercise	Calories	Distance	Time

Water Intake ______________

Cooldown ______________

Feeling ☆ ☆ ☆ ☆ ☆

Notes

Today's Goal _______________________ Ⓜ Ⓣ Ⓦ Ⓣ Ⓕ **S** **S**

Muscle Group Focus _______________________ Weight _______ Date/Time _______

Stretch ◯   Warm-Up _______________________

Strength Training

Exercise		Set 1	Set 2	Set 3	Set 4	Set 5	Set 6
	Reps						
	Weight						
	Reps						
	Weight						
	Reps						
	Weight						
	Reps						
	Weight						
	Reps						
	Weight						
	Reps						
	Weight						
	Reps						
	Weight						
	Reps						
	Weight						
	Reps						
	Weight						

Cardio

Exercise	Calories	Distance	Time

Water Intake _______________________

Cooldown _______________________

Feeling ☆ ☆ ☆ ☆ ☆

Notes

Today's Goal

Muscle Group Focus ______________________ Weight ______ Date/Time ______

Stretch ◯   Warm-Up ______________________

Strength Training

Exercise		Set 1	Set 2	Set 3	Set 4	Set 5	Set 6
	Reps						
	Weight						
	Reps						
	Weight						
	Reps						
	Weight						
	Reps						
	Weight						
	Reps						
	Weight						
	Reps						
	Weight						
	Reps						
	Weight						
	Reps						
	Weight						
	Reps						
	Weight						

Cardio

Exercise	Calories	Distance	Time

Water Intake ______________

Cooldown ______________

Feeling ☆ ☆ ☆ ☆ ☆

Notes

Today's Goal

$\quad$ M T W T F **S** **S**

Muscle Group Focus $\quad$ Weight $\quad$ Date/Time

Stretch ◯ $\quad$ Warm-Up

Strength Training

Exercise		Set 1	Set 2	Set 3	Set 4	Set 5	Set 6
	Reps						
	Weight						
	Reps						
	Weight						
	Reps						
	Weight						
	Reps						
	Weight						
	Reps						
	Weight						
	Reps						
	Weight						
	Reps						
	Weight						
	Reps						
	Weight						
	Reps						
	Weight						

Cardio

Exercise	Calories	Distance	Time

Water Intake

Cooldown

Feeling ☆ ☆ ☆ ☆ ☆

Notes

Today's Goal

Muscle Group Focus ___________________ Weight _______ Date/Time _________

Stretch ◯   Warm-Up ____

Strength Training

Exercise		Set 1	Set 2	Set 3	Set 4	Set 5	Set 6
	Reps						
	Weight						
	Reps						
	Weight						
	Reps						
	Weight						
	Reps						
	Weight						
	Reps						
	Weight						
	Reps						
	Weight						
	Reps						
	Weight						
	Reps						
	Weight						
	Reps						
	Weight						

Cardio

Exercise	Calories	Distance	Time

Water Intake _________________

Cooldown _________________

Feeling ☆ ☆ ☆ ☆ ☆

Notes

Today's Goal

M T W T F **S** **S**

Muscle Group Focus ______________________ Weight ______ Date/Time ______

Stretch ○   Warm-Up ______________________

Strength Training

Exercise		Set 1	Set 2	Set 3	Set 4	Set 5	Set 6
	Reps						
	Weight						
	Reps						
	Weight						
	Reps						
	Weight						
	Reps						
	Weight						
	Reps						
	Weight						
	Reps						
	Weight						
	Reps						
	Weight						
	Reps						
	Weight						
	Reps						
	Weight						

Cardio

Exercise	Calories	Distance	Time

Water Intake ______________________

Cooldown ______________________

Feeling ☆ ☆ ☆ ☆ ☆

Notes

Today's Goal

Muscle Group Focus   Weight   Date/Time

Stretch ◯   Warm-Up

Strength Training

Exercise		Set 1	Set 2	Set 3	Set 4	Set 5	Set 6
	Reps						
	Weight						
	Reps						
	Weight						
	Reps						
	Weight						
	Reps						
	Weight						
	Reps						
	Weight						
	Reps						
	Weight						
	Reps						
	Weight						
	Reps						
	Weight						
	Reps						
	Weight						
	Reps						
	Weight						

Cardio

Exercise	Calories	Distance	Time

Water Intake

Cooldown

Feeling ☆ ☆ ☆ ☆ ☆

Notes

Today's Goal ___________________________ Ⓜ Ⓣ Ⓦ Ⓣ Ⓕ **Ⓢ** **Ⓢ**

Muscle Group Focus ___________________ Weight ______ Date/Time ______

Stretch ◯ Warm-Up ___________________________________

Strength Training

Exercise		Set 1	Set 2	Set 3	Set 4	Set 5	Set 6
	Reps						
	Weight						
	Reps						
	Weight						
	Reps						
	Weight						
	Reps						
	Weight						
	Reps						
	Weight						
	Reps						
	Weight						
	Reps						
	Weight						
	Reps						
	Weight						
	Reps						
	Weight						
	Reps						
	Weight						

Cardio

Exercise	Calories	Distance	Time

Water Intake ___________________

Cooldown ___________________

Feeling ☆ ☆ ☆ ☆ ☆

Notes

Today's Goal

(M) (T) (W) (T) (F) (S) (S)

Muscle Group Focus ___________________   Weight _______   Date/Time _______

Stretch ◯   Warm-Up ____

Strength Training

Exercise		Set 1	Set 2	Set 3	Set 4	Set 5	Set 6
	Reps						
	Weight						
	Reps						
	Weight						
	Reps						
	Weight						
	Reps						
	Weight						
	Reps						
	Weight						
	Reps						
	Weight						
	Reps						
	Weight						
	Reps						
	Weight						
	Reps						
	Weight						

Cardio

Exercise	Calories	Distance	Time

Water Intake ___________________

Cooldown ___________________

Feeling ☆ ☆ ☆ ☆ ☆

Notes

Today's Goal ___________________________ Ⓜ Ⓣ Ⓦ Ⓣ Ⓕ ⬤S ⬤S

Muscle Group Focus ___________________ Weight ________ Date/Time ________

Stretch ◯   Warm-Up ___________________________

Strength Training

Exercise		Set 1	Set 2	Set 3	Set 4	Set 5	Set 6
	Reps						
	Weight						
	Reps						
	Weight						
	Reps						
	Weight						
	Reps						
	Weight						
	Reps						
	Weight						
	Reps						
	Weight						
	Reps						
	Weight						
	Reps						
	Weight						
	Reps						
	Weight						

Cardio

Exercise	Calories	Distance	Time

Water Intake ___________________

Cooldown ___________________

Feeling ☆ ☆ ☆ ☆ ☆

Notes

Today's Goal

M T W T F **S** **S**

Muscle Group Focus ___________________ Weight _______ Date/Time _______

Stretch ◯ Warm-Up ___________________________

Strength Training

Exercise		Set 1	Set 2	Set 3	Set 4	Set 5	Set 6
	Reps						
	Weight						
	Reps						
	Weight						
	Reps						
	Weight						
	Reps						
	Weight						
	Reps						
	Weight						
	Reps						
	Weight						
	Reps						
	Weight						
	Reps						
	Weight						
	Reps						
	Weight						
	Reps						
	Weight						

Cardio

Exercise	Calories	Distance	Time

Water Intake ___________________

Cooldown ___________________

Feeling ☆ ☆ ☆ ☆ ☆

Notes

Today's Goal

(M) (T) (W) (T) (F) (S) (S)

Muscle Group Focus ______________________ Weight ______ Date/Time ______

Stretch ○   Warm-Up ______________________

Strength Training

Exercise		Set 1	Set 2	Set 3	Set 4	Set 5	Set 6
	Reps						
	Weight						
	Reps						
	Weight						
	Reps						
	Weight						
	Reps						
	Weight						
	Reps						
	Weight						
	Reps						
	Weight						
	Reps						
	Weight						
	Reps						
	Weight						
	Reps						
	Weight						

Cardio

Exercise	Calories	Distance	Time

Water Intake ______________________

Cooldown ______________________

Feeling ☆ ☆ ☆ ☆ ☆

Notes

Today's Goal

(M) (T) (W) (T) (F) (S) (S)

Muscle Group Focus ____________________ Weight ________ Date/Time __________

Stretch ◯   Warm-Up ____

Strength Training

Exercise		Set 1	Set 2	Set 3	Set 4	Set 5	Set 6
	Reps						
	Weight						
	Reps						
	Weight						
	Reps						
	Weight						
	Reps						
	Weight						
	Reps						
	Weight						
	Reps						
	Weight						
	Reps						
	Weight						
	Reps						
	Weight						
	Reps						
	Weight						

Cardio

Exercise	Calories	Distance	Time

Water Intake ____________

Cooldown ____________

Feeling ☆ ☆ ☆ ☆ ☆

Notes

Today's Goal ___________________________   M T W T F **S** **S**

Muscle Group Focus ___________________   Weight _______   Date/Time _______

Stretch ◯   Warm-Up ___________________

Strength Training

Exercise		Set 1	Set 2	Set 3	Set 4	Set 5	Set 6
	Reps						
	Weight						
	Reps						
	Weight						
	Reps						
	Weight						
	Reps						
	Weight						
	Reps						
	Weight						
	Reps						
	Weight						
	Reps						
	Weight						
	Reps						
	Weight						
	Reps						
	Weight						

Cardio

Exercise	Calories	Distance	Time

Water Intake ___________________

Cooldown ___________________

Feeling ☆ ☆ ☆ ☆ ☆

Notes

Today's Goal

(M) (T) (W) (T) (F) **S** **S**

Muscle Group Focus ______________________ Weight ______ Date/Time ______

Stretch ○   Warm-Up ________________________________

Strength Training

Exercise		Set 1	Set 2	Set 3	Set 4	Set 5	Set 6
	Reps						
	Weight						
	Reps						
	Weight						
	Reps						
	Weight						
	Reps						
	Weight						
	Reps						
	Weight						
	Reps						
	Weight						
	Reps						
	Weight						
	Reps						
	Weight						
	Reps						
	Weight						
	Reps						
	Weight						

Cardio

Exercise	Calories	Distance	Time

Water Intake ________________

Cooldown ________________

Feeling ☆ ☆ ☆ ☆ ☆

Notes

Today's Goal ___________________________ Ⓜ Ⓣ Ⓦ Ⓣ Ⓕ ⬤S ⬤S

Muscle Group Focus ___________________ Weight ______ Date/Time ______

Stretch ◯   Warm-Up ___________________________

Strength Training

Exercise		Set 1	Set 2	Set 3	Set 4	Set 5	Set 6
	Reps						
	Weight						
	Reps						
	Weight						
	Reps						
	Weight						
	Reps						
	Weight						
	Reps						
	Weight						
	Reps						
	Weight						
	Reps						
	Weight						
	Reps						
	Weight						
	Reps						
	Weight						
	Reps						
	Weight						

Cardio

Exercise	Calories	Distance	Time

Water Intake ___________________

Cooldown ___________________

Feeling ☆ ☆ ☆ ☆ ☆

Notes

Today's Goal

Ⓜ Ⓣ Ⓦ Ⓣ Ⓕ ● ●

Muscle Group Focus ________________________ Weight ______ Date/Time ______

Stretch ◯   Warm-Up ________________________

Strength Training

Exercise		Set 1	Set 2	Set 3	Set 4	Set 5	Set 6
	Reps						
	Weight						
	Reps						
	Weight						
	Reps						
	Weight						
	Reps						
	Weight						
	Reps						
	Weight						
	Reps						
	Weight						
	Reps						
	Weight						
	Reps						
	Weight						
	Reps						
	Weight						

Cardio

Exercise	Calories	Distance	Time

Water Intake ______

Cooldown ______

Feeling ☆ ☆ ☆ ☆ ☆

Notes

Today's Goal

(M)(T)(W)(T)(F)(**S**)(**S**)

Muscle Group Focus ___________________________   Weight _______   Date/Time _______

Stretch ◯   Warm-Up _______________________________________

Strength Training

Exercise		Set 1	Set 2	Set 3	Set 4	Set 5	Set 6
	Reps						
	Weight						
	Reps						
	Weight						
	Reps						
	Weight						
	Reps						
	Weight						
	Reps						
	Weight						
	Reps						
	Weight						
	Reps						
	Weight						
	Reps						
	Weight						
	Reps						
	Weight						
	Reps						
	Weight						

Cardio

Exercise	Calories	Distance	Time

Water Intake _______________

Cooldown _______________

Feeling ☆ ☆ ☆ ☆ ☆

Notes

Today's Goal

M T W T F **S** **S**

Muscle Group Focus _______________ Weight _______ Date/Time _______

Stretch ◯   Warm-Up _______________

Strength Training

Exercise		Set 1	Set 2	Set 3	Set 4	Set 5	Set 6
	Reps						
	Weight						
	Reps						
	Weight						
	Reps						
	Weight						
	Reps						
	Weight						
	Reps						
	Weight						
	Reps						
	Weight						
	Reps						
	Weight						
	Reps						
	Weight						
	Reps						
	Weight						

Cardio

Exercise	Calories	Distance	Time

Water Intake _______________

Cooldown _______________

Feeling ☆ ☆ ☆ ☆ ☆

Notes

Today's Goal _______________________   Ⓜ Ⓣ Ⓦ Ⓣ Ⓕ ⬤S ⬤S

Muscle Group Focus _____________________   Weight _______   Date/Time _______

Stretch ◯   Warm-Up _______________________

Strength Training

Exercise		Set 1	Set 2	Set 3	Set 4	Set 5	Set 6
	Reps						
	Weight						
	Reps						
	Weight						
	Reps						
	Weight						
	Reps						
	Weight						
	Reps						
	Weight						
	Reps						
	Weight						
	Reps						
	Weight						
	Reps						
	Weight						
	Reps						
	Weight						

Cardio

Exercise	Calories	Distance	Time

Water Intake _______________

Cooldown _______________

Feeling ☆ ☆ ☆ ☆ ☆

Notes

Today's Goal

M T W T F **S** **S**

Muscle Group Focus ___________________________   Weight _______   Date/Time _______

Stretch ◯   Warm-Up ___________________________

Strength Training

Exercise		Set 1	Set 2	Set 3	Set 4	Set 5	Set 6
	Reps						
	Weight						
	Reps						
	Weight						
	Reps						
	Weight						
	Reps						
	Weight						
	Reps						
	Weight						
	Reps						
	Weight						
	Reps						
	Weight						
	Reps						
	Weight						
	Reps						
	Weight						
	Reps						
	Weight						

Cardio

Exercise	Calories	Distance	Time

Water Intake ___________________________

Cooldown ___________________________

Feeling ☆ ☆ ☆ ☆ ☆

Notes

Today's Goal

M T W T F **S** **S**

Muscle Group Focus ___________________________ Weight ________ Date/Time __________

Stretch ◯   Warm-Up ______________________________________

Strength Training

Exercise		Set 1	Set 2	Set 3	Set 4	Set 5	Set 6
	Reps						
	Weight						
	Reps						
	Weight						
	Reps						
	Weight						
	Reps						
	Weight						
	Reps						
	Weight						
	Reps						
	Weight						
	Reps						
	Weight						
	Reps						
	Weight						
	Reps						
	Weight						

Cardio

Exercise	Calories	Distance	Time

Water Intake ____________________

Cooldown ____________________

Feeling ☆ ☆ ☆ ☆ ☆

Notes

Today's Goal   (M) (T) (W) (T) (F) (S) (S)

Muscle Group Focus _______________________ Weight _______ Date/Time _______

Stretch ◯   Warm-Up _______________________

Strength Training

Exercise		Set 1	Set 2	Set 3	Set 4	Set 5	Set 6
	Reps						
	Weight						
	Reps						
	Weight						
	Reps						
	Weight						
	Reps						
	Weight						
	Reps						
	Weight						
	Reps						
	Weight						
	Reps						
	Weight						
	Reps						
	Weight						
	Reps						
	Weight						
	Reps						
	Weight						

Cardio

Exercise	Calories	Distance	Time

Water Intake _______________________

Cooldown _______________________

Feeling ☆ ☆ ☆ ☆ ☆

Notes

Today's Goal ___________________ Ⓜ Ⓣ Ⓦ Ⓣ Ⓕ ⬤S ⬤S

Muscle Group Focus ________________________ Weight ______ Date/Time ______

Stretch ◯   Warm-Up ___________________________________

Strength Training

Exercise		Set 1	Set 2	Set 3	Set 4	Set 5	Set 6
	Reps						
	Weight						
	Reps						
	Weight						
	Reps						
	Weight						
	Reps						
	Weight						
	Reps						
	Weight						
	Reps						
	Weight						
	Reps						
	Weight						
	Reps						
	Weight						
	Reps						
	Weight						

Cardio

Exercise	Calories	Distance	Time

Water Intake ___________________

Cooldown ___________________

Feeling ☆ ☆ ☆ ☆ ☆

Notes

Today's Goal

M T W T F S S

Muscle Group Focus _______________________ Weight ________ Date/Time __________

Stretch ◯   Warm-Up ________________________________

Strength Training

Exercise		Set 1	Set 2	Set 3	Set 4	Set 5	Set 6
	Reps						
	Weight						
	Reps						
	Weight						
	Reps						
	Weight						
	Reps						
	Weight						
	Reps						
	Weight						
	Reps						
	Weight						
	Reps						
	Weight						
	Reps						
	Weight						
	Reps						
	Weight						

Cardio

Exercise	Calories	Distance	Time

Water Intake __________

Cooldown __________

Feeling ☆ ☆ ☆ ☆ ☆

Notes

Today's Goal

(M) (T) (W) (T) (F) (S) (S)

Muscle Group Focus __________________________ Weight _________ Date/Time _________

Stretch ◯   Warm-Up _______________________________

Strength Training

Exercise		Set 1	Set 2	Set 3	Set 4	Set 5	Set 6
	Reps						
	Weight						
	Reps						
	Weight						
	Reps						
	Weight						
	Reps						
	Weight						
	Reps						
	Weight						
	Reps						
	Weight						
	Reps						
	Weight						
	Reps						
	Weight						
	Reps						
	Weight						

Cardio

Exercise	Calories	Distance	Time

Water Intake _______________

Cooldown _______________

Feeling ☆ ☆ ☆ ☆ ☆

Notes

Today's Goal

M T W T F S S

Muscle Group Focus ___________________ Weight ________ Date/Time ________

Stretch ◯ Warm-Up ___________________

Strength Training

Exercise		Set 1	Set 2	Set 3	Set 4	Set 5	Set 6
	Reps						
	Weight						
	Reps						
	Weight						
	Reps						
	Weight						
	Reps						
	Weight						
	Reps						
	Weight						
	Reps						
	Weight						
	Reps						
	Weight						
	Reps						
	Weight						
	Reps						
	Weight						
	Reps						
	Weight						

Cardio

Exercise	Calories	Distance	Time

Water Intake ___________________

Cooldown ___________________

Feeling ☆ ☆ ☆ ☆ ☆

Notes

Today's Goal

Today's Goal ___________________________ M T W T F **S** **S**

Muscle Group Focus ___________________ Weight _______ Date/Time _______

Stretch ◯   Warm-Up _______________________________

Strength Training

Exercise		Set 1	Set 2	Set 3	Set 4	Set 5	Set 6
	Reps						
	Weight						
	Reps						
	Weight						
	Reps						
	Weight						
	Reps						
	Weight						
	Reps						
	Weight						
	Reps						
	Weight						
	Reps						
	Weight						
	Reps						
	Weight						
	Reps						
	Weight						
	Reps						
	Weight						

Cardio

Exercise	Calories	Distance	Time

Water Intake _______________

Cooldown _______________

Feeling ☆ ☆ ☆ ☆ ☆

Notes

Today's Goal

Today's Goal _______________________ (M) (T) (W) (T) (F) **(S)** **(S)**

Muscle Group Focus _______________________ Weight _______ Date/Time _______

Stretch ◯   Warm-Up _______________________

Strength Training

Exercise		Set 1	Set 2	Set 3	Set 4	Set 5	Set 6
	Reps						
	Weight						
	Reps						
	Weight						
	Reps						
	Weight						
	Reps						
	Weight						
	Reps						
	Weight						
	Reps						
	Weight						
	Reps						
	Weight						
	Reps						
	Weight						
	Reps						
	Weight						
	Reps						
	Weight						

Cardio

Exercise	Calories	Distance	Time

Water Intake _______________________

Cooldown _______________________

Feeling ☆ ☆ ☆ ☆ ☆

Notes

Today's Goal ________________   Ⓜ Ⓣ Ⓦ Ⓣ Ⓕ **Ⓢ** **Ⓢ**

Muscle Group Focus ________________   Weight ______   Date/Time ______

Stretch ◯   Warm-Up ________________

Strength Training

Exercise		Set 1	Set 2	Set 3	Set 4	Set 5	Set 6
	Reps						
	Weight						
	Reps						
	Weight						
	Reps						
	Weight						
	Reps						
	Weight						
	Reps						
	Weight						
	Reps						
	Weight						
	Reps						
	Weight						
	Reps						
	Weight						
	Reps						
	Weight						
	Reps						
	Weight						

Cardio

Exercise	Calories	Distance	Time

Water Intake ________________

Cooldown ________________

Feeling ☆ ☆ ☆ ☆ ☆

Notes

Today's Goal

M T W T F **S** **S**

Muscle Group Focus ______________________ Weight ________ Date/Time ________

Stretch ◯   Warm-Up ______________________

Strength Training

Exercise		Set 1	Set 2	Set 3	Set 4	Set 5	Set 6
	Reps						
	Weight						
	Reps						
	Weight						
	Reps						
	Weight						
	Reps						
	Weight						
	Reps						
	Weight						
	Reps						
	Weight						
	Reps						
	Weight						
	Reps						
	Weight						
	Reps						
	Weight						
	Reps						
	Weight						

Cardio

Exercise	Calories	Distance	Time

Water Intake ____________

Cooldown ____________

Feeling ☆ ☆ ☆ ☆ ☆

Notes

Today's Goal

M T W T F S S

Muscle Group Focus ___________________ Weight _______ Date/Time _________

Stretch ◯   Warm-Up _______________________________________

Strength Training

Exercise		Set 1	Set 2	Set 3	Set 4	Set 5	Set 6
	Reps						
	Weight						
	Reps						
	Weight						
	Reps						
	Weight						
	Reps						
	Weight						
	Reps						
	Weight						
	Reps						
	Weight						
	Reps						
	Weight						
	Reps						
	Weight						
	Reps						
	Weight						

Cardio

Exercise	Calories	Distance	Time

Water Intake _______________

Cooldown _______________

Feeling ☆ ☆ ☆ ☆ ☆

Notes

Today's Goal

Muscle Group Focus ________________________ Weight ________ Date/Time ________

M T W T F S S

Stretch ◯   Warm-Up ________________________

Strength Training

Exercise		Set 1	Set 2	Set 3	Set 4	Set 5	Set 6
	Reps						
	Weight						
	Reps						
	Weight						
	Reps						
	Weight						
	Reps						
	Weight						
	Reps						
	Weight						
	Reps						
	Weight						
	Reps						
	Weight						
	Reps						
	Weight						
	Reps						
	Weight						
	Reps						
	Weight						

Cardio

Exercise	Calories	Distance	Time

Water Intake ________

Cooldown ________

Feeling ☆ ☆ ☆ ☆ ☆

Notes

Today's Goal

M T W T F **S** **S**

Muscle Group Focus ___________________________ Weight ________ Date/Time ________

Stretch ◯   Warm-Up ___________________________

Strength Training

Exercise		Set 1	Set 2	Set 3	Set 4	Set 5	Set 6
	Reps						
	Weight						
	Reps						
	Weight						
	Reps						
	Weight						
	Reps						
	Weight						
	Reps						
	Weight						
	Reps						
	Weight						
	Reps						
	Weight						
	Reps						
	Weight						
	Reps						
	Weight						

Cardio

Exercise	Calories	Distance	Time

Water Intake ___________________________

Cooldown ___________________________

Feeling ☆ ☆ ☆ ☆ ☆

Notes

Today's Goal

M T W T F S S

Muscle Group Focus ________________________ Weight ________ Date/Time ________

Stretch ◯   Warm-Up ________________________

Strength Training

Exercise		Set 1	Set 2	Set 3	Set 4	Set 5	Set 6
	Reps						
	Weight						
	Reps						
	Weight						
	Reps						
	Weight						
	Reps						
	Weight						
	Reps						
	Weight						
	Reps						
	Weight						
	Reps						
	Weight						
	Reps						
	Weight						
	Reps						
	Weight						

Cardio

Exercise	Calories	Distance	Time

Water Intake ________________________

Cooldown ________________________

Feeling ☆ ☆ ☆ ☆ ☆

Notes

Today's Goal

M T W T F **S** **S**

Muscle Group Focus ___________________________ Weight _______ Date/Time _______

Stretch ◯   Warm-Up ___________________________

Strength Training

Exercise		Set 1	Set 2	Set 3	Set 4	Set 5	Set 6
	Reps						
	Weight						
	Reps						
	Weight						
	Reps						
	Weight						
	Reps						
	Weight						
	Reps						
	Weight						
	Reps						
	Weight						
	Reps						
	Weight						
	Reps						
	Weight						
	Reps						
	Weight						

Cardio

Exercise	Calories	Distance	Time

Water Intake ___________________________

Cooldown ___________________________

Feeling ☆ ☆ ☆ ☆ ☆

Notes

Today's Goal

M T W T F **S** **S**

Muscle Group Focus ______________________ Weight ______ Date/Time ______

Stretch ○   Warm-Up ______________________

Strength Training

Exercise		Set 1	Set 2	Set 3	Set 4	Set 5	Set 6
	Reps						
	Weight						
	Reps						
	Weight						
	Reps						
	Weight						
	Reps						
	Weight						
	Reps						
	Weight						
	Reps						
	Weight						
	Reps						
	Weight						
	Reps						
	Weight						
	Reps						
	Weight						

Cardio

Exercise	Calories	Distance	Time

Water Intake ______________

Cooldown ______________

Feeling ☆ ☆ ☆ ☆ ☆

Notes

CPSIA information can be obtained
at www.ICGtesting.com
Printed in the USA
LVHW051112170321
681672LV00023B/1906